Mastering Makeup: A Comprehensive Guide To Application Techniques

Angela Ramos

Published by Angela Ramos, 2024.

While every precaution has been taken in the preparation of this book, the publisher assumes no responsibility for errors or omissions, or for damages resulting from the use of the information contained herein.

MASTERING MAKEUP: A COMPREHENSIVE GUIDE TO APPLICATION TECHNIQUES

First edition. July 11, 2024.

ISBN: 979-8227580832

Written by Angela Ramos.

Table of Contents

To all the makeup artists who transform faces into canvases and to everyone who finds confidence and joy in makeup this is for you with love.

Title: Mastering Makeup: A Comprehensive Guide to Application Techniques

Introduction:

Welcome to "Mastering Makeup," your ultimate guide to mastering various makeup application techniques. Whether you're a beginner or an experienced makeup enthusiast, these techniques are insightful and helpful. This ebook will cover a wide range of makeup application techniques, from the basics of creating a flawless base to the complexities of contouring, highlighting, and mastering eyeshadow looks and blending. We will cover everything you need to know to elevate your makeup game. Each chapter is designed to provide clear, step-by-step instructions and helpful tips and tricks to help you achieve professional-level results.

Makeup is more than just a way to enhance one's appearance; it's a form of self-expression, creativity, and empowerment. With the right tools, techniques, and knowledge, anyone can achieve stunning makeup looks that reflect their personality and style. Whether you're getting ready for a special event, experimenting with new trends, or simply looking to elevate your everyday makeup routine, "Mastering Makeup" has you covered. So grab your brushes, prepare your makeup kit, and embark on this journey together to unlock your full makeup potential.

Let's master the makeup techniques to help everyone confidently achieve their desired looks. I'm here to guide you through each step of the process to help you understand the how and why of makeup. Let's begin our journey to mastering makeup!

Chapter 1: Color Theory

- Color theory plays a crucial role in mastering makeup as it helps individuals understand how different hues interact and how they can enhance natural beauty or create specific looks. Here's how color theory applies to mastering makeup:

UNDERSTANDING UNDERTONES:

○ Everyone has skin undertones, which can be warm, cool, or neutral. Knowing your undertone helps you select makeup products that match your skin tone, such as foundation and concealer. Warm undertones pair well with peachy or golden hues, while cool undertones suit shades with blue or pink undertones.

Color Correction:

○ Color theory guides the use of color correctors to neutralize specific skin concerns. For instance, green correctors can counteract redness, while peach or orange correctors can conceal dark circles or hyperpigmentation.

Creating Harmony:

○ Applying makeup involves creating harmony among different colors used on the face. This includes coordinating eyeshadow shades with lipstick colors and blush tones to achieve a cohesive and balanced look.

Contrast and Emphasis:

○ By understanding complementary colors, makeup artists can create contrast and emphasis. For example, using complementary colors on the eyes can make them pop, while applying a lipstick shade that contrasts with the eye makeup can draw attention to the lips.

Color Wheel Techniques:

○ Makeup artists often refer to the color wheel to create various makeup looks. Techniques like monochromatic, analogous, or triadic color schemes can achieve different effects, whether a subtle, harmonious look or a bold, artistic statement.

Personalization:

○ While understanding color theory principles is essential, it's also important to experiment and personalize makeup looks according to individual preferences and features. What works for one person may not work for another, so adapting color theory principles to suit personal style is critical.

A solid grasp of color theory empowers individuals to make informed decisions about product selection, application techniques, and overall makeup looks, resulting in polished, professional results tailored to individual beauty.

Chapter 2: The Art of Blending

———

- Understanding the Importance of Blending: Learn why blending is crucial in achieving seamless and natural-looking makeup.

BLENDING MAKEUP IS crucial because it ensures a seamless and natural look, prevents harsh lines or patches, and helps the makeup last longer. Proper blending creates a smooth transition between shades and textures, enhancing the overall appearance and providing a polished finish.

- Blending Techniques: Explore different blending techniques for foundation, concealer, blush, and eyeshadow to achieve flawless results.

Blending techniques are essential for achieving a flawless makeup application. Here are some blending techniques for foundation, concealer, blush, and eyeshadow:

Foundation:

○ Makeup Sponge: A damp makeup sponge, such as the Beautyblender, helps achieve a seamless, airbrushed finish by bouncing and blending foundation into the skin.

○ Flat-Top Kabuki Brush: Dense and flat-topped brushes are ideal for buffing liquid or cream foundation into the skin, providing an even flawless application.

Concealer:

○ Precision Concealer Brush: A small, tapered brush allows for the precise application of concealer to target areas like blemishes or dark circles and helps blend the product seamlessly.

○ Makeup Sponge: A small makeup sponge or the pointed tip of a giant sponge can also blend concealer, especially under the eyes.

Blush:

○ Fluffy Blush Brush: Opt for a soft, fluffy brush with rounded edges to apply and blend powder blush onto the cheeks. The fluffy bristles help diffuse the color for a natural-looking flush.

○ Duo Fiber Brush: Combined with synthetic and natural bristles, Duo fiber brushes are great for applying cream or liquid blushes. They blend effortlessly and prevent streakiness.

Eyeshadow:

○ Eyeshadow Blending Brush: A soft, fluffy blending brush with tapered bristles is essential for seamlessly blending eyeshadow in the crease and creating smooth transitions between colors.

○ Flat Eyeshadow Brush: Use a flat, dense brush to pack eyeshadow onto the lid, ensuring intense color payoff before blending with a blending brush.

General Tools:

○ Makeup Sponge: Aside from foundation and concealer, makeup sponges can blend cream contour, highlighter, and even powder products for a soft, diffused finish.

○ Clean Fingers: Sometimes, using clean fingers can be the most effective tool for blending certain products, especially cream or liquid formulas.

When selecting brushes and tools, consider the type of makeup products you use most frequently and your personal blending preferences. Investing in high-quality tools can yield better results and make blending more enjoyable. You should also regularly clean your brushes and tools to maintain their performance and prevent bacterial buildup.

● Practice Exercises: Follow step-by-step exercises to hone your blending skills and perfect your technique.

Regular blending techniques are vital in improving your makeup skills and achieving flawless results. Here are some step-by-step exercises to help you hone your blending skills:

Foundation Blending:

○ Step 1: Start with a freshly cleansed and moisturized face.

○ Step 2: Apply a small amount of liquid foundation to the back of your hand or directly onto your face.

○ Step 3: Pick the foundation with your preferred tool (makeup sponge or brush).

○ Step 4: Begin blending the foundation onto your skin, starting from the center of your face and working outward in gentle, tapping or swirling motions.

○ Step 5: Pay special attention to areas where you need more coverage, such as around the nose or on blemishes.

○ Step 6: Take your time to ensure the foundation is seamlessly blended into your skin with no harsh lines or streaks.

Concealer Application:

○ Step 1: After applying foundation, dot concealer under your eyes in a triangular shape and on any areas that need extra coverage, such as blemishes or redness.

○ Step 2: Use a small concealer brush or your finger to gently blend the concealer into your skin, using tapping or patting motions.

○ Step 3: Continue blending until the concealer seamlessly merges with your foundation, providing a smooth and even finish.

○ Step 4: Set the concealer with a translucent powder to prevent creasing and increase longevity.

Blush Blending:

○ Step 1: Smile to locate the apples of your cheeks.

○ Step 2: Use a blush brush to pick up a small amount of blush powder or cream.

○ Step 3: Apply the blush to the apples of your cheeks in a circular motion, blending upwards towards your temples.

○ Step 4: Blend out any harsh lines using a clean makeup sponge or a clean brush.

○ Step 5: Repeat the process if you want to build up the intensity of the blush, ensuring seamless blending between layers.

Eyeshadow Blending:

○ Step 1: Apply an eyeshadow primer or light base to your eyelids to create a smooth canvas.

○ Step 2: Choose a transition shade slightly darker than your skin tone and apply it to the crease using a fluffy blending brush.

○ Step 3: Use windshield wiper motions to blend the transition shade back and forth in the crease until it's seamlessly diffused.

○ Step 4: Apply a deeper shade to the outer corner of the eye and blend it into the crease using small, circular motions.

○ Step 5: Use a clean blending brush to soften harsh lines and seamlessly transition between colors.

○ Step 6: Repeat the process with additional eyeshadow colors, gradually increasing the intensity and blending each shade as you go.

Practice Makes Perfect:

○ Set aside dedicated time to practice your blending skills regularly.

○ Experiment with different techniques, tools, and makeup products to find what works best for you.

○ Don't be afraid to make mistakes—they're essential to learning. Note what works and what doesn't, and adjust your technique accordingly.

○ Watch makeup tutorials and follow along to learn new blending techniques from makeup artists and beauty influencers.

By incorporating these exercises into your makeup routine and dedicating time to practice regularly, you'll gradually improve your blending skills and achieve professional-looking results.

Chapter 3: Mastering Contouring

- What is Contouring?: Understand the concept of contouring and how it can enhance your facial features.

CONTOURING IS A MAKEUP technique that enhances and sculpts facial features by creating shadows and highlights. It involves using slightly darker and lighter makeup products than your natural skin tone to create the illusion of more defined cheekbones, a slimmer nose, a more pronounced jawline, and other desired facial contours.

Here's how contouring typically works:

○ **Preparation**: Start with a clean, moisturized face. Apply your foundation as usual to create an even base.

○ **Choosing Products**: You'll need a contour product a few shades darker than your natural skin tone and a highlighter a few shades lighter. Depending on your preference, these can come in cream, powder, or stick form.

○ **Identifying Areas to Contour**: Common areas to contour include the hollows of the cheeks, along the jawline, the sides of the nose, and the temples. You can also contour the forehead to make it appear smaller and under the chin to create the illusion of a more defined jawline.

○ **Application:** Use a contour brush, sponge, or fingers to apply the darker shade along the areas you want to define. Blend well to avoid harsh lines.

○ **Highlighting**: Apply the lighter shade to the high points of your face where light naturally hits, such as the tops of the cheekbones, the bridge of the nose, the brow bone, and the cupid's bow above the lips. This helps to accentuate these features.

○ **Blending**: Blend the contour and highlight together seamlessly to avoid harsh lines. This is crucial for achieving a natural-looking finish.

○ **Setting**: Set your makeup with a translucent powder to ensure it stays in place throughout the day.

Contouring can be a subtle enhancement for everyday makeup or more dramatic for special occasions or photography. Practicing and finding the right balance for your face shape and personal style is essential. Different face shapes may also require different contouring techniques to achieve the desired effect. Contouring is a versatile makeup technique that can help accentuate your best features and create a more sculpted appearance.

- Choosing the Right Products: Learn how to select the appropriate contouring products for your skin tone and face shape.

Selecting the right contouring products is essential for achieving a natural, flattering look that complements your skin tone and face shape. Here's how to choose the appropriate contouring products:

○ **Consider Your Skin Tone**: When choosing a contour shade, opt for a color only a few shades darker than your natural skin tone. Avoid shades that are too warm or cool, as they can look unnatural on your skin. Choose a contour shade with a cool undertone if you have fair skin. A contour shade with a warm undertone may work best for medium to deep skin tones.

○ **Choose the Right Formula**: Contouring products come in various formulas, including creams, powders, and sticks. Choose a formula based on your skin type and personal preference. Creams are ideal for dry skin as they provide a dewy finish and blend seamlessly into the skin. Powders are suitable for oily or combination skin as they offer a matte finish and help control shine. Stick formulas are convenient for on-the-go touch-ups and provide buildable coverage.

○ **Consider Your Face Shape**: Different face shapes require different contouring techniques and products to achieve the desired effect. Here are some general guidelines:

○ **Round Face**: Use a contour shade to create shadows along the sides of the face to add definition and slim down the appearance. Focus on contouring the outer edges of the forehead, the hollows of the cheeks, and along the jawline.

○ **Square Face**: Soften the angles of a square face by contouring the corners of the forehead, the jawline, and the sides of the face. Focus on creating more rounded contours to balance out the sharpness of the face shape.

    ○ **Heart-Shaped Face**: Contour the sides of the forehead and temples to minimize the width of the top of the face. Apply contour along the sides of the jawline to soften its appearance. Highlight the center of the forehead and chin to balance out the broader forehead and narrower chin.

    ○ **Oval Face**: An oval face shape is already well-balanced, so focus on enhancing your natural features rather than altering the shape. Contour the hollows of the cheeks, the sides of the nose, and the jawline for added definition.

○ **Test Products Before Purchasing:** Swatch a contouring product on your jawline or inner wrist to ensure it matches your skin tone and blends seamlessly. Try products in-store or look for samples to test before committing to a full-size product.

By considering your skin tone, face shape, and personal preferences, you can choose contouring products that enhance your features and create a beautifully sculpted look.

    ● Contouring Techniques: Explore different contouring techniques for sculpting the cheeks, nose, jawline, and forehead.

Contouring allows you to sculpt various facial features to enhance your natural bone structure. Here are different contouring techniques for sculpting the cheeks, nose, jawline, and forehead:

- **Cheeks:**

  - To define the hollows of your cheeks, suck in your cheeks to locate the natural indentation.

  - Apply a contour shade directly into the hollows using a contour brush, starting from the hairline towards the corners of your mouth.

  - Blend the contour shade upward and outward using a blending brush or sponge. Make sure to blend well to avoid harsh lines.

- **Note:**

  - To slim and define the nose, apply a thin line of contour shade on each side of the nose using a small, angled brush.

  - Start the contour shade from the beginning of the eyebrows and extend it down towards the tip of the nose.

  - Blend the contour shade using a blending brush or sponge, focusing on diffusing the edges to create a seamless transition.

- **Jawline:**

○ To create a more defined jawline, apply contour shade along the jawline using a contour brush or angled brush.

○ Start from the earlobes and blend the contour shade downwards towards the chin, following the natural curve of your jawline.

○ Blend the contour shade well to avoid harsh lines and ensure a natural-looking finish.

○ **Forehead**:

○ To minimize the appearance of a more prominent forehead, apply contour shade along the hairline using a contour brush or powder brush.

○ Start from the temples and blend the contour shade towards the center of the forehead, focusing on the outer edges.

○ Blend the contour shade well into the hairline to avoid any visible lines.

Remember, blending is critical to achieving a natural-looking contour. Use a blending brush or sponge to blend the contour shades seamlessly into your skin for a flawless finish. Additionally, practice makes perfect, so don't be afraid to experiment with different techniques and products to find what works best for your face shape and desired look.

● Tips for a Natural Look: Discover tips and tricks for achieving a natural-looking contour that complements your features.

Achieving a natural-looking contour is all about subtlety and blending. Here are some tips and tricks for achieving a contour that complements your features while maintaining a natural appearance:

○ **Choose the Right Shade**: Opt for a contour shade that is only slightly darker than your natural skin tone. Avoid shades that are too warm or cool, as they can appear unnatural on the skin.

○ **Blend, Blend, Blend**: Blending is crucial for creating a natural-looking contour. Use a blending brush or sponge to blend the contour shade seamlessly into your skin, focusing on diffusing harsh lines or edges.

○ **Less is More**: Start with a small amount of product and build it up gradually. Adding more than removing excess product once it's applied is easier.

○ **Focus on Key Areas**: Rather than contouring your entire face, focus on critical areas that will enhance your natural bone structure, such as the hollows of the cheeks, the sides of the nose, the jawline, and the temples.

○ **Use a Light Hand**: Apply contour product with a light hand to avoid applying too much product simultaneously. Tap off any excess product from your brush before applying it to your face.

○ **Blend with Foundation**: After applying your contour shade, blend it further by gently patting the contoured areas with your foundation brush or sponge. This helps to soften the edges further and blend the contour seamlessly into your foundation.

○ **Natural Lighting**: Apply your contour in natural lighting whenever possible to ensure the most natural-looking result. Artificial lighting can sometimes distort colors and make your contour appear more intense than it is.

○ **Practice Makes Perfect**: Contouring is a skill that takes practice to master. Take the time to experiment with different techniques and products to find what works best for your face shape and skin tone.

Following these tips and tricks, you can achieve a natural-looking contour that enhances your features without looking overly done or heavy. Remember to take your time and blend thoroughly for the best results.

- Advanced Contouring: Dive into advanced contouring techniques for more dramatic and defined looks.

Advanced contouring techniques allow you to create more dramatic and defined looks by strategically sculpting and shaping your facial features. Here are some advanced contouring techniques to achieve a more dramatic effect:

Cream Contouring and Layering:

○ Start with a cream contour product a few shades darker than your skin tone. Apply it to the areas you want to define, such as the hollows of the cheeks, the sides of the nose, the jawline, and the forehead.

○ Use a cream highlighter a few shades lighter than your skin tone to accentuate the high points of your face, such as the tops of the cheekbones, the bridge of the nose, the brow bone, and the cupid's bow.

○ Layer powder contour and highlight products on top of the cream products to intensify the contour and highlight, creating a more defined and sculpted look.

○ Blend each layer thoroughly to ensure a seamless transition between the cream and powder products.

Contouring with Multiple Shades:

○ Use multiple shades of contour to create depth and dimension on your face. Start with a lighter contour shade to map out the areas you want to define, then layer a darker shade to intensify the shadows.

○ For example, you can use a lighter contour shade to contour the hollows of the cheeks and a darker shade to deepen the contour along the jawline and temples.

○ Blend the multiple contour shades seamlessly to create a natural gradient effect.

Nose Contouring Techniques:

○ Experiment with different nose contouring techniques to reshape and define your nose.

○ Use a combination of contour and highlight shades to create the illusion of a slimmer or more straight nose.

○ For example, you can contour the sides of the nose to make it appear slimmer and use a highlight shade down the center of the nose to make it appear straighter and more defined.

○ Blend the contour and highlight shades carefully to avoid harsh lines or edges.

Precision Contouring:

○ Use smaller brushes and precise application techniques to sculpt specific areas of your face more accurately.

○ For example, use a small, angled brush to contour the jawline and chin for a sharper and more defined look.

○ Focus on blending the contour shades seamlessly into your skin to create a natural-looking finish, even with precise application.

Contouring for Photography or Stage:

○ If you're contouring for photography or stage performances, you may need to apply contour products more heavily to ensure they appear well under bright lights or camera flashes.

○ Experiment with contour products with stronger pigmentation and buildable coverage to achieve the desired intensity.

○ Blend carefully to avoid harsh lines or uneven patches, as these can be more noticeable in photographs or under stage lighting.

These advanced contouring techniques require practice and experimentation, but they can help you achieve more dramatic and defined looks for special occasions, performances, or photoshoots. Mix thoroughly and customize the techniques to suit your face shape and personal style.

Chapter 4: The Power of Highlighting

- The Purpose of Highlighting: Learn how highlighting can add dimension and luminosity to your complexion.

HIGHLIGHTING IS A MAKEUP technique that adds dimension, luminosity, and glow to the complexion by accentuating the high points of the face where light naturally hits. Here's how highlighting can enhance your overall look:

○ **Enhances Facial Structure**: Highlighting helps accentuate and define the face's natural contours. By applying highlighter to specific areas, such as the tops of the cheekbones, the brow bone, the bridge of the nose, and the cupid's bow above the lips, you can create the illusion of more prominent features and a sculpted appearance.

○ **Adds Luminosity**: Highlighter contains light-reflecting particles that can give the skin a radiant and luminous glow. When applied to the high points of the face, highlighter catches and reflects light, making those areas appear brighter and more illuminated. This can help to create a youthful and healthy-looking complexion.

○ **Creates Depth and Dimension**: When paired with contouring, highlighters help contrast the face, adding depth and dimension. While contouring creates shadows to define specific areas, highlighting brings forward other areas by attracting light to them. Together, contouring and highlighting work harmoniously to sculpt and shape the face for a more balanced and symmetrical appearance.

○ **Provides a Healthy Glow**: Highlighting can give the skin a natural, lit-from-within glow. Whether you prefer a subtle, dewy look or a more intense, high-shine finish, a highlighter can help to create a healthy and radiant complexion that looks youthful and fresh.

○ **Complements Makeup Looks**: Highlighting is versatile and can be incorporated into various makeup looks to enhance the overall effect. Whether you're going for a natural, everyday look or a glamorous, full-face makeup look, adding a touch of highlighter can elevate your makeup and give it that extra oomph.

○ **Boosts Confidence**: Highlighting can help to boost confidence by accentuating your best features and enhancing your natural beauty. Feeling good about your appearance can positively impact your mood and overall self-confidence.

In summary, highlighting is a makeup technique that adds dimension, luminosity, and glow to the complexion by accentuating the high points of the face. Whether aiming for a subtle, natural look or a more intense, glamorous effect, highlighting can help you achieve a radiant and youthful complexion that enhances your overall appearance.

● Selecting the Right Highlighter: Explore different types of highlighters and how to choose the best one for your skin type and desired finish.

Selecting the right highlighter is crucial for achieving your desired makeup look while considering your skin type and desired finish. Here are different types of highlighters and tips on how to choose the best one for you:

○ **Powder Highlighter**:

○ Ideal for: All skin types, especially oily or combination skin.

○ Features: Powder highlighters typically come in pressed powder form and offer a wide range of shades and finishes, from subtle to intense.

○ How to choose: If you have oily skin, opt for a finely milled powder highlighter with a matte or satin finish to avoid adding excess shine. Choose a powder highlighter with a creamy texture for dry or mature skin or infused with hydrating ingredients to prevent it from looking dry or cakey on the skin.

○ **Cream Highlighter**:

○ Ideal for: Dry or mature skin types.

○ Features: Cream highlighters have a creamy texture that blends seamlessly into the skin, providing a natural-looking glow. They often come in pots, sticks, or tubes.

○ How to choose: Look for cream highlighters with a lightweight and non-greasy formula that won't emphasize texture or fine lines. Opt for shades that complement your skin tone for a more natural finish, or go for a more pigmented shade for a more intense glow.

○ **Liquid Highlighter:**

○ Ideal for: All skin types, especially dry or mature skin.

○ Features: Liquid highlighters come in fluid form and can be mixed with foundation or applied directly to the skin for a luminous finish. They provide a dewy and natural-looking glow.

○ How to choose: Choose a liquid highlighter with a lightweight and buildable formula that can be customizable to your desired level of intensity. Look for shades that complement your skin tone and have light-reflecting particles to enhance your complexion.

○ **Stick Highlighter:**

○ Ideal for: All skin types, especially dry or mature skin.

○ Features: Stick highlighters come in a stick or crayon form, making them convenient for on-the-go applications. They have a creamy texture that blends easily into the skin for a natural-looking glow.

○ Choose a stick highlighter with a creamy, blendable formula that glides smoothly onto the skin without tugging or pulling. Opt for shades complement your skin tone and provide a luminous finish without emphasizing texture or fine lines.

○ **Baked Highlighter**:

○ Ideal for: All skin types.

○ Features: Baked highlighters are made by baking liquid or cream formulas until they solidify into a powder. They often have a velvety texture and offer a high-shine finish.

○ How to choose: Look for baked highlighters with a smooth and buttery texture that blends effortlessly onto the skin. Choose shades that complement your skin tone and provide a radiant glow without looking glittery or chunky.

When selecting a highlighter, consider your skin type, desired finish, and preference for the application method. Experiment with different formulas, shades, and textures to find the perfect highlighter that enhances your natural beauty and complements your overall makeup look.

● Highlighting Techniques: Discover various highlighting techniques for accentuating the high points of your face, such as the cheekbones, brow bone, and cupid's bow.

Highlighting techniques can help accentuate the high points of your face, bringing light to specific areas for a radiant and glowing complexion. Here are various highlighting techniques for accentuating different regions of the face:

○ **Cheekbones**:

○ Apply highlighter to the tops of your cheekbones to add dimension and glow to your face.

○ Use a small, fluffy brush or a fan brush to apply the highlighter sweepingly along the highest points of your cheekbones.

○ Start from the outer edge of your eye and blend the highlighter towards your temples for a natural-looking glow.

○ You can also apply a highlighter slightly above your blush for extra radiance.

○ **Brow Bone**:

○ Highlighting the brow bone can help lift the eyes and create the illusion of more enormous, awake eyes.

○ Use a small, precise brush or your fingertips to apply highlighter to the brow bone just beneath the arch of your eyebrow.

○ Blend the highlighter downwards towards the tail of your brow and upwards towards the inner corner of your eye.

○ Be sure to blend well to avoid any harsh lines or patches.

○ **Cupid's Bow:**

○ Highlighting the cupid's bow can accentuate your lips and make them appear fuller.

○ Use a small, precise brush or your fingertips to apply highlighter to the cupid's bow, which is the dip in the center of your upper lip.

○ Apply the highlighter sparingly to avoid overemphasizing this area.

○ Blend the highlighter gently to soften any harsh edges.

○ **Bridge of the Nose:**

○ Highlighting the bridge of the nose can create the illusion of a taller, more defined nose.

○ Use a small, precise brush or a sponge to apply highlighter in a thin line down the center of your nose.

○ Start from between your eyebrows and blend the highlighter downwards towards the tip of your nose.

○ Be careful not to apply too much product, making your nose appear oily or exaggerated.

○ **Inner Corner of the Eyes:**

○ Highlighting the inner corner of the eyes can brighten and open up your eyes, giving you a more awake and refreshed appearance.

○ Use a small, precise brush or your fingertips to apply highlighter to the inner corners of your eyes.

○ Apply the highlighter sparingly to avoid any fallout or irritation.

○ Blend the highlighter gently to soften harsh edges and create a seamless transition.

When applying highlighter, remember to blend well to achieve a natural-looking glow. Experiment with different techniques and placement to find what works best for your face shape and desired makeup look. Whether you prefer a subtle, lit-from-within glow or a more intense, high-shine finish, highlighting can help you achieve a radiant complexion that enhances your natural beauty.

● Tips for a Radiant Glow: Learn tips and tricks for achieving a radiant and dewy finish with your highlighter application.

Achieving a radiant and dewy finish with your highlighter application can elevate your makeup look and give your complexion a healthy glow. Here are some tips and tricks for achieving that coveted radiant glow:

○ **Prep Your Skin**:

○ Start with a well-moisturized and hydrated base. Apply a hydrating primer or moisturizer to ensure your skin is smooth and plump, which will help the highlighter blend seamlessly and adhere better.

○ **Choose the Right Highlighter**:

○ Opt for a highlighter with a luminous or dewy finish to achieve a radiant glow. Cream, liquid, or stick highlighters provide a more natural-looking radiance than powders.

○ Look for highlighters with finely milled shimmer particles that catch the light without emphasizing texture or pores.

○ **Apply Strategically**:

○ Focus on applying highlighter to the high points of your face where light naturally hits, such as the tops of the cheekbones, the brow bone, the cupid's bow, the bridge of the nose, and the inner corners of the eyes.

○ Use a light hand and build up the intensity gradually. It's easier to add more product than to remove excess.

○ For a radiant finish, concentrate the highlighter on the areas you want to glow, but avoid applying it all over your face to prevent looking overly shiny.

○ **Blend Well:**

○ Blend the highlighter seamlessly into your skin using a damp makeup sponge, a fluffy brush, or fingertips. Softly blend the edges to avoid any harsh lines or patches.

○ For cream or liquid highlighters, pat and press the product into your skin rather than rubbing it to maintain its luminosity and prevent your foundation from moving underneath.

○ **Layer for Intensity:**

○ For a more intense glow, layer different formulas of highlighters. Start with a cream or liquid highlighter as a base, then set it with a powder highlighter in a similar shade for added luminosity and longevity.

○   Layering highlighters can create a multidimensional effect and enhance the overall radiance of your complexion.

○ **Set with Setting Spray:**

○ After applying your highlighter, lightly mist your face with a setting spray to meld all the makeup layers together and create a seamless finish. This will help lock in the glow and ensure it lasts throughout the day.

○ **Highlight Your Body:**

○ Don't forget to highlight other body parts, such as the collarbones, shoulders, and décolletage, for an all-over radiant glow. This can enhance the overall luminosity of your look, especially for special occasions or when wearing outfits that reveal more skin.

By following these tips and tricks, you can achieve a radiant and dewy finish with your highlighter application, enhancing your natural beauty and giving your complexion a healthy glow that lasts all day.

- Customizing Your Highlight: Experiment with shades and textures to customize your highlight for various occasions and looks.

Customizing your highlight allows you to tailor your glow to suit different occasions, makeup looks, and personal preferences.

Here's how you can experiment with various shades and textures to customize your highlight:

Shades:

○ Explore a variety of highlighter shades to find the ones that complement your skin tone and desired makeup look.

○ Champagne or golden shades are flattering and work well for most skin tones. They provide a warm, luminous glow that is perfect for everyday wear.

○ Rose gold or peachy shades: These shades add a hint of warmth and color to the skin, giving you a fresh and radiant complexion. They are great for adding a subtle pop of color to your highlight.

○ Pearl or icy shades: These shades have cool undertones and create a striking, frosty effect on the skin. They are perfect for achieving a dramatic and ethereal glow, especially for evening or special occasions.

○ Mix different highlighter shades to create your custom shade that complements your skin tone and enhances your overall makeup look.

Textures:

○ Try different highlighter textures to achieve varying levels of intensity and luminosity.

○ Powder highlighters are the most common type and come in various finishes, from subtle shimmer to intense metallic. They are easy to blend and provide buildable coverage that allows you to control the intensity of your glow.

○ Cream or liquid highlighters: These formulas offer a more natural-looking radiance and provide a dewy, lit-from-within glow. They are perfect for a fresh and youthful complexion, especially for dry or mature skin.

○ Balm or jelly highlighters: These innovative formulas have a bouncy texture that melts into the skin, providing a sheer, glossy finish. They are great for creating a natural, "wet" look that mimics the appearance of healthy, hydrated skin.

○ Experiment with layering different textures together to create a multidimensional effect. For example, you can layer a cream highlighter underneath a powder highlighter to intensify the glow and prolong its wear time.

Occasions and Looks:

○ Tailor your highlight to suit the occasion and the makeup look you're going for.

○ Opt for a subtle, natural-looking highlight that enhances your features without overpowering them for everyday wear. Choose shades complementing your skin tone and providing a soft, luminous glow.

○ For special occasions or evening looks, feel free to amp up the intensity of your highlight for a more dramatic effect. Experiment with brighter shades, metallic finishes, and layering techniques to create a show-stopping glow that catches the light and turns heads.

By experimenting with different shades and textures, you can customize your highlights to suit your style, enhance your natural beauty, and create a radiant glow that complements any occasion or makeup look. Don't be afraid to get creative and have fun with your highlighter application!

Chapter 5: Eyeshadow Mastery

-

- Understanding Eyeshadow Basics: Learn about different finishes, textures, and formulations.

UNDERSTANDING EYESHADOW basics, including finishes, textures, and formulations, is essential for creating beautiful eye makeup looks. Here's an overview of each aspect:

○ **Finishes**:

○ **Matte**: Matte eyeshadows have a flat, non-reflective finish. They are great for adding depth and definition to the eyes and are commonly used in crease and transition shades.

○ **Shimmer**: Shimmer eyeshadows contain fine particles that reflect light, giving them a soft, luminous finish. They add dimension and brightness to the eyes and highlight the lid or inner corner.

○ **Metallic**: Metallic eyeshadows have a high-shine finish with intense pigmentation. They provide a foil-like effect on the lids and are often used to create bold and glamorous eye looks.

○ **Satin**: Satin eyeshadows have a subtle sheen that falls between matte and shimmer finishes. They offer a soft, luminous effect without being too sparkly and are versatile for both everyday and special occasion looks.

○ **Glitter**: Glitter eyeshadows contain larger particles of glitter that provide a high-impact, sparkly finish. They are perfect for adding drama and glamour to eye makeup, especially for evening or festive occasions.

○ **Textures**:

○ **Powder**: Powder eyeshadows are the most common and versatile type of eyeshadow. They come in various finishes, including matte, shimmer, metallic, and satin, and can be easily blended for seamless application.

○ **Cream**: Cream eyeshadows have a creamy texture that glides smoothly onto the lids. They offer intense pigmentation and are long-lasting, making them great for creating bold and vibrant eye looks. Cream eyeshadows can be applied with fingers or brushes and are often used as a base for powder eyeshadows to enhance their color payoff and longevity.

○ **Pressed**: Pressed eyeshadows come in a compact palette and have a firm, pressed consistency. They are convenient for travel and on-the-go touch-ups and offer buildable coverage for customizable looks.

○ **Loose**: Loose eyeshadows consist of finely milled pigment that is loose in a jar or container. They provide intense color payoff and can be applied wet or dry for different effects. Loose eyeshadows require careful application to prevent fallout and can be messy, but they offer unparalleled vibrancy and shine.

○ **Formulations**:

○ **Traditional**: Traditional eyeshadows come in pans or compacts and can be powder- or cream-based. They are versatile, easy to use, and suitable for beginners and experienced makeup enthusiasts.

○ **Liquid**: Liquid eyeshadows have a liquid formulation and come in tubes or wand applicators. They provide intense pigmentation and long-lasting wear, perfect for creating graphic or bold eye looks. Liquid eyeshadows often dry to a matte or metallic finish and can be layered for added intensity.

○ **Pencil**: Eyeshadow pencils are convenient and portable, perfect for on-the-go applications. They come in various finishes, including matte, shimmer, and metallic, and can be used as eyeliner or eyeshadow for versatile looks.

Understanding different eyeshadow finishes, textures, and formulations allows you to choose the right products for your desired makeup looks and preferences. An eyeshadow type is perfect whether you prefer a soft and natural eye makeup look or a bold and dramatic statement.

- Eyeshadow Application Techniques: Explore step-by-step tutorials for applying eyeshadow to achieve various eye looks, including natural, smoky, and colorful.

Certainly! Here are step-by-step tutorials for achieving different eyeshadow looks:

○ **Natural Eye Look**:

Step 1: Prime your eyelids with an eyeshadow primer to ensure longevity and vibrant color payoff.

Step 2: Apply a neutral matte eyeshadow that matches your skin tone all over your eyelids as a base. This will help create a seamless canvas for other eyeshadows.

Step 3: Choose a medium-toned matte eyeshadow slightly darker than your skin tone. Apply it to the crease of your eyelids using a fluffy blending brush, focusing on windshield wiper motions to blend it evenly.

Step 4: Apply a lighter shimmer eyeshadow shade to the inner corners of your eyes and the center of your eyelids. This will add brightness and dimension to your eyes.

Step 5: Optionally, apply a soft brown or taupe eyeshadow along the lower lash line to add definition.

Step 6: Finish the look with mascara on your upper and lower lashes for a natural, polished finish.

○ **Smoky Eye Look**:

Step 1: Prime your eyelids to ensure your eyeshadow stays in place throughout the day and intensifies the colors.

Step 2: Use a small, dense brush to apply matte eyeshadow in a dark shade, such as black, charcoal, or deep brown, to the outer corner of your eyelids.

Step 3: Blend the dark eyeshadow into the crease using a fluffy blending brush, focusing on creating between the dark shade and your skin tone.

Step 4: Apply a medium-toned eyeshadow, such as a deep plum or navy, to the center of your eyelids and blend it into the dark shade to create depth and dimension.

Step 5: Use a lighter shimmer eyeshadow shade and apply it to the inner corners of your eyes and the center of your eyelids to add brightness and highlight.

Step 6: Combine the same dark eyeshadow along the lower lash line for a cohesive look.

Step 7: Apply eyeliner along the upper lash line and waterline, and coat your lashes with mascara for added drama.

○ **Colorful Eye Look**:

Step 1: Prime your eyelids to ensure a vibrant color payoff and prevent creasing.

Step 2: Apply a transition shade, such as a light brown or peach, to the crease of your eyelids using a fluffy blending brush to create a smooth transition between colors.

Step 3: Choose a bold, colorful eyeshadow and apply it to the outer corner of your eyelids using a dense brush, packing on the color for maximum intensity.

Step 4: Blend the colorful eyeshadow into the crease and towards the inner corner of your eyes using a clean blending brush, ensuring a seamless transition between colors.

Step 5: Using a flat eyeshadow brush, apply a complementary or contrasting color to the center of your eyelids, blending it into the other colors for a gradient effect.

Step 6: Use a lighter shimmer eyeshadow shade and apply it to the inner corners of your eyes and the center of your eyelids to add brightness and dimension.

Step 7: Optionally, add a pop of color along the lower lash line to tie the look together.

Step 8: Finish with eyeliner along the upper lash line and waterline, and coat your lashes with mascara to complete the colorful eye look.

Remember to blend your eyeshadows well for a seamless and polished finish, and don't be afraid to experiment with different colors, textures, and techniques to create your desired eye look.

- Blending Like a Pro: Master blending eyeshadows seamlessly for professional-looking eye makeup.

Mastering the art of blending eyeshadows seamlessly is essential for achieving professional-looking eye makeup. Here are some tips and techniques to help you mix like a pro:

○ **Start with a Clean Canvas**:

  ○ Begin by applying an eyeshadow primer or a concealer to your eyelids. This will create a smooth base for your eyeshadows to adhere to and help prolong their wear time.

○ **Use the Right Tools**:

  ○ Invest in high-quality eyeshadow brushes with soft, fluffy bristles designed for blending.

  ○ A blending brush with a tapered or dome-shaped tip is ideal for diffusing and blending eyeshadows seamlessly.

○ **Choose the Right Eyeshadow Formulas**:

  ○ Opt for eyeshadows with buildable and blendable formulas that are easy to work with.

  ○ Matte eyeshadows are great for creating depth and dimension in the crease, while shimmer or metallic shades can be applied to the lid or inner corner to add brightness and dimension.

  ○ Cream eyeshadows can be used as a base or applied directly to the lid for a more intense color payoff.

○ **Start with Transition Shades:**

○ Begin by applying a transition shade, a matte eyeshadow slightly darker than your skin tone, into the crease using a blending brush.

○ Use the windshield wiper and small circular motions to blend the transition shade back and forth along the crease until it is diffused and seamless.

○ **Layer and Build Color Gradually:**

○ Layer eyeshadows gradually, starting with lighter shades and building to darker ones.

○ Use a light hand and apply eyeshadows in small amounts, blending as you go to prevent harsh lines and ensure a smooth transition between colors.

○ **Work in Layers:**

○ Work in layers by applying and blending one eyeshadow at a time.

○ Start with the lightest shade as a base, then gradually build up the intensity with darker shades, focusing on the outer corner and crease of the eye.

○ **Blend, Blend, Blend:**

○ Blend each eyeshadow thoroughly to ensure a seamless transition between colors.

○ Use back-and-forth windshield wipers and small circular motions to blend eyeshadows seamlessly.

○ Blend the edges of each eyeshadow to soften any harsh lines and create a gradient effect.

○ **Use a Clean Brush for Diffusing**:

○ Keep a clean blending brush on hand to diffuse and blend out any harsh lines or edges as needed.

○ Use this clean brush to soften and blend the edges of your eyeshadows for a polished finish.

○ **Practice Patience and Practice**:

○ Achieving a perfectly blended eyeshadow look takes time and practice, so don't rush the process.

○ Experiment with different techniques and products to find what works best for you, and feel free to make mistakes.

Following these tips and techniques, you can master blending eyeshadows seamlessly for professional-looking eye makeup that enhances natural beauty. Practice patience, experiment with different colors and textures, and have fun with your eyeshadow looks!

- Enhancing Eye Shape: Discover techniques for enhancing your eye shape with eyeshadow, including how to make eyes appear larger or more lifted.

Enhancing your eye shape with eyeshadow can help create the illusion of more enormous, more lifted eyes. Here are some techniques to achieve this:

- **Make Eyes Appear Larger:**

  ○ Start by applying a light, matte, or eyeshadow base over the eyelid to create a bright, open base.

  ○ To add brightness and make the eyes appear more awake, use light, shimmery eyeshadow, or highlighter on the inner corner of the eyes.

  ○ Apply a medium-toned eyeshadow shade to the crease and blend upwards towards the brow bone. This creates the illusion of depth and dimension, making the eyes appear more prominent.

  ○ Avoid using dark eyeshadows on the eyelid, as they can make the eyes look smaller. Instead, focus on using lighter shades to open up the eyes.

- **Create a Winged Eyeliner Effect:**

  ○ Use eyeshadow to create a winged eyeliner effect, making the eyes appear more lifted.

  ○ Start by applying a medium-toned eyeshadow to the outer corner of the eye, extending it slightly upwards and outwards towards the end of the eyebrow.

○ Use a small, angled brush to blend and soften the eyeshadow, creating a winged shape that lifts the eyes.

○ You can also use a darker eyeshadow shade or eyeliner to intensify the winged effect.

- **Highlight the Brow Bone:**

  ○ Apply a light, shimmery eyeshadow or highlighter to the brow bone to lift and define the eyebrows.

  ○ Use a small eyeshadow brush to apply the highlighter directly under the brow's arch, blending downwards towards the eyelid.

  ○ This technique lifts the face and draws attention to the eyes, making them appear larger and more defined.

- **Focus on the Lower Lash Line:**

  ○ Apply a light, shimmery eyeshadow or highlighter to the inner corner of the lower lash line to brighten and open up the eyes.

  ○ Use a medium-toned eyeshadow shade to softly define the lower lash line, focusing on the outer corner and blending towards the center.

  ○ Avoid using dark eyeshadows on the lower lash line, as they can make the eyes appear smaller. Instead, stick to lighter shades to enhance the eyes.

- **Curl Your Lashes and Apply Mascara:**

  ○ Use an eyelash curler to curl your lashes before applying mascara. This helps to lift and open up the eyes, making them appear larger.

  ○ Apply several coats of lengthening or volumizing mascara to the upper and lower lashes to enhance the eye shape and make them appear more defined.

By incorporating these techniques into your eyeshadow application, you can enhance your eye shape and create the illusion of more enormous, more lifted eyes. Experiment with different shades, textures, and techniques to find what works best for your eye shape and desired look.

- **Troubleshooting:** Learn how to troubleshoot common eyeshadow mistakes and how to fix them for flawless results.

Troubleshooting common eyeshadow mistakes is essential for achieving flawless results in your eye makeup. Here are some common mistakes and how to fix them:

Patchy or Uneven Application:

  ○ **Cause:** This can occur due to using too much or too little, uneven blending, or applying eyeshadow over a dry base.

○ **Solution**: Start by applying an eyeshadow primer or concealer to create a smooth base for your eyeshadows. Then, use a light hand and build up the eyeshadow gradually, blending as you go. Blend the edges thoroughly to avoid any harsh lines or patches. If the eyeshadow still appears patchy, use a clean blending brush to soften and blend out any uneven areas.

Fallout Under the Eyes:

○ **Cause**: Fallout occurs when excess eyeshadow falls onto the under-eye area during application, leaving smudges or streaks.

○ **Solution**: Tap off any excess eyeshadow from your brush before applying it to your eyelids. You can also hold a tissue or makeup shield under your eyes to catch any fallout. If fallout occurs, use a clean makeup brush or wipe to gently sweep away the excess eyeshadow without smudging your makeup.

Muddy or Overblended Eyeshadow:

○ **Cause**: Blending can cause the colors to mix and appear muddy or indistinct.

○ **Solution**: Be mindful of how much you blend your eyeshadows and avoid overblending. Use a light hand and blend in small, controlled motions to maintain the clarity and intensity of each shade. If the eyeshadows become muddy, use a clean blending brush to diffuse the colors and soften any harsh edges.

Harsh Lines or Edges:

○ **Cause**: Harsh lines or edges can occur when eyeshadows are not appropriately blended, or the wrong brush is used.

○ **Solution**: Use a clean blending brush to blend out any harsh lines or edges and soften the eyeshadows for a seamless finish. You can also use a transition shade to help blend out the edges and create a smooth transition between colors. Alternatively, gently use a makeup sponge or cotton swab to smudge and soften harsh lines.

Creasing or Fading Throughout the Day:

○ **Cause**: Creasing and fading can occur when using eyeshadows that are not long-wearing or when applying them over a greasy or oily base.

○ **Solution**: Use an eyeshadow primer or concealer to create a smooth, oil-free base for your eyeshadows. This will help prevent creasing and fading and prolong the wear time of your eye makeup. You can also set your eyeshadow with a translucent setting powder to lock it in place and prevent it from creasing throughout the day.

By troubleshooting these common eyeshadow mistakes and implementing the suggested solutions, you can achieve flawless eye makeup results and confidently create stunning looks. Practice patience and experiment with different techniques to find what works best for you.

Conclusion:

Mastering makeup is a journey of self-expression, creativity, and confidence. This ebook explored the fundamentals of makeup application, from skincare preparation to advanced techniques for enhancing natural beauty. We delved into the world of understanding undertones and selecting the right products for your unique features.

Congratulations! You've completed "Mastering Makeup," and you're now equipped with the knowledge and skills to master various makeup application techniques. As you continue to practice and experiment with different styles, methods, and products, embrace the joy of discovery and self-expression. Confidence is your ultimate accessory, whether aiming for a natural everyday look or a glamorous evening ensemble.

Remember, practice makes perfect, so don't be afraid to experiment and have fun with your makeup. With dedication and perseverance, you'll be able to achieve any makeup look you desire. Thank you for embarking on this journey with us. May your makeup skills continue to evolve, empowering you to express yourself fearlessly and beautifully. Here's to embracing your unique beauty and mastering the art of makeup! Happy glamming!

Don't miss out!

Visit the website below and you can sign up to receive emails whenever Angela Ramos publishes a new book. There's no charge and no obligation.

https://books2read.com/r/B-A-LIORB-LVJPD

BOOKS 2 READ

Connecting independent readers to independent writers.

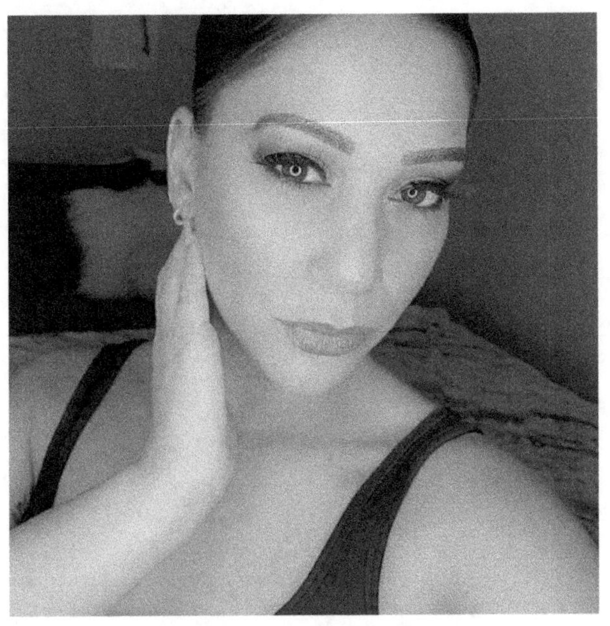

About the Author

As a child, I fell in love with makeup. I converted that passion into a profession, becoming a certified freelance makeup artist. Having done this for 8+ years, I've helped clients feel and look beautiful. Each client is seen and treated as a work of art.

www.ingramcontent.com/pod-product-compliance
Lightning Source LLC
Chambersburg PA
CBHW052128150726
48002CB00006B/2532